MENIERE MAN
AND THE FILM DIRECTOR

THE SELF-HELP BOOK FOR MENIERE'S VERTIGO

PAGE ADDIE
UNITED KINGDOM AND AUSTRALIA

ISBN: 978-0-9876270-0-1 BIC Subject category: VFJB A catalogue record for this book is available from Bowkers. 1. vertigo 2. dizziness. 3. dizzy. 4. meniere's disease. 5. meniere 6. inner ear. 7. vestibular. 9. vertigo. 10 causes of vertigo. 11. imbalance. 12. what is vertigo. 13 low salt. 14 coping with vertigo.

This is what amazon readers are saying:

This book helped give me the desire to get on with life. For 2 years I have been afraid to do many things. I may be more cautious of what I do, I can say I am now trying to do them. Thanks it was a great book.

-C.D

Great read for Meniere's disease. Very good tools to help you deal MD on a daily basis.

-J.N

The author shares his experience in a very clear, detailed and easily understood manner. This book is essential to anyone suffering with vertigo.

-M.L

Reading this book, it won't take you many pages to realize that the man who wrote it knows EXACTLY what he is talking about.

-D.R

The author has done a tremendous job of writing a book that includes what's necessary to cope with even the worst attack of vertigo.

-E.S

It is an inspirational book.

-C.L

CONTENT

Preface

This 3rd edition of *Meniere Man and the Movie Director* and *Vertigo Vertigo* is revised and updated with features such as the new Anti-Vertigo Notebook, which includes 40 Ways To Help Yourself Get Over Meniere's Vertigo, plus ground breaking self-help strategies for coping and managing each stage of a vertigo attack. This book is now titled *Meniere Man 'The Self Help Book for Meniere's Vertigo*.

MENIERE MAN AND THE FILM DIRECTOR

In the movie Vertigo, Alfred Hitchcock, a famous film director, stranded his characters on the edge of a cataclysm. You may not have seen the movie, but as a Meniere sufferer you'll certainly know what real vertigo is.

Vertigo is one of the more dynamic and frightening symptoms of Meniere's disease. Vertigo is the sensation of horizontal or rotational spinning, lasting between thirty minutes to an hour or for many hours. Each time you have an attack, you are thrown over the edge, into the cataclysm of rotational spinning vertigo. And it's not a psychological thriller. It's a reality horror story. Spontaneous vertigo can happen at any time, any place. The unpredictable nature of vertigo is why you feel constantly on edge.

When you have Meniere's disease, unfortunately you'll have a history which involves episodes of true whirling vertigo. If you're anything like me, the first vertigo attack is the one you remember in detail. The attack would have sent you and your family rushing off to see the doctor.

Words like dreadful, awful, terrible could never describe an attack. Meniere's vertigo symptoms defy description.

You most probably turned up at the Doctor's surgery gripping hold of your friend's arm. The doctor would have noted: *showing significant physical and mental distress, looked pale and sweaty. On medical examination vital signs show elevated blood pressure, rapid pulse, nystagmus. Patient breathing faster than normal.*

All you would have been thinking is, quick, give me a shot of something to make it stop! If you were lucky the doctor would have given you an injection of stemetil and the symptoms would have subsided. Later your doctor would have arranged for you to see an Otolaryngologist. After reading the hearing test results and listening to my history of recent dizziness, my specialist cleared his throat, took a deep breath and said, "You've got Meniere's disease. It is an extremely aggressive condition that medical science knows little about."

I asked the obvious question. "What is Meniere's?" He went on to explain: Fluctuating hearing loss (sometimes good or bad). Episodic vertigo (can be violent). Tinnitus or ringing in the ears (usually low tone roaring). Aural fullness (pressure, discomfort). And it's incurable."

Severe shock! An incurable disease. People had labelled me with a few names before, incorrigible, yes, but never incurable. Always the optimist, I still asked the question. "Can I recover from this?" And I got the following answer. "As I have said before, it is incurable, but the outcome is variable, since the disease pattern of exacerbation and remission makes evaluation of treatment and prognosis difficult to predict. My best advice right now is to go home and rest. Cut down on salt and keep away from stress. And here's a prescription for stemetil and betahistine."

At that point I thought ?!

Keep away from stress? Not possible! I

was very stressed out sitting in his surgery. Still the eternal optimist, I asked, "I have organized a family skiing trip, do you think I should go?" "Sure, life is short. Go out and enjoy yourself." His last remark puzzled more than anything he had told me! Maybe it was the way he said it?

Well, I did go to the mountain the following weekend, with a medical stamp of approval. And the sky was blue. The powder was fresh. And Meniere's was left behind, or so I thought. I was a newbie at this point. On the way home I had to stop driving. I just lay on the back seat for the six hour winding mountain road trip home. Yet that journey made me realize that even with Meniere's disease, I could still do life. For me, getting out there when I could, became part of the cure for this incurable optimist.

A month later a friend was arriving from Canada to go fishing. I didn't cancel him out, I continued with the plan to go sea fishing and then travel by car to a remote river to fly fish in the wilderness. I did wonder if I was capable of going on such an adventure. But all it took was a new focus and the company of a good friend. I was lucky and I didn't have any attacks.

So again rather than have a calendar of cancelled plans and empty days, I decided that living with Meniere's was going to be about taking a positive approach to living life.

When you have Meniere's disease it's not easy to find a life within it. Especially in the early days of diagnosis when the stress of vertigo attacks is unrelenting. You are unable to recuperate from one attack to the next. It is overwhelming because there seems to be no pattern to these attacks. The threat of a vertigo attack makes you stay in a state of readiness and your mind constantly sends panic messages to your body. Even the slightest feeling of dizziness puts you on high alert.

The fact is when you have been diagnosed with Meniere's disease, you are certainly going to have repeated attacks of vertigo. How you cope is a personal choice. Many Meniere's sufferers are driven to radical surgery in order to get relief from vertigo. Some people cope in ways that others would not contemplate.

Vincent Van Gogh, the Impressionist painter, who is thought to have had Meniere's, placed himself in and out of institutions and struggled to a point of causing himself physical damage, by removing the offending ear!

Personally, I managed Meniere's vertigo, by initially taking prescribed medication. Then I took an alternative holistic self-help management approach in order minimize and eliminate vertigo completely.

I am proof that working towards getting better as soon as you can, using personal management techniques, will enhance your chances of stopping vertigo altogether. What I figured out is this; you simply can't afford to wait until you feel better. You must start to move in the direction of wellness immediately in order to get over Meniere's.

The first step is to look at yourself as a whole person. You already have a lot going for you. Your arms, hands, legs, stomach, back, heart, lungs, bones, muscles and mind, are not affected by Meniere's. It is only one part of your body that malfunctions some of the time.

What I advocate is using the time between vertigo attacks to work on your general health and coping strategies. When you get fitter, stronger and healthier, you will find you cope better with vertigo attacks.

There are many ways you can do this. From changing your diet, to reducing stress, to doing more exercise, practicing meditation, taking medication, using supplements and applying cognitive thinking techniques.

This is what I did and it worked. Getting a life back with Meniere's doesn't just happen. For me, the greatest healer is the self. It does take some personal inner strength to get through rough days. This is what I want to share with you: how to help yourself and recover a full and active life. If I can do it, so can you.

VERTIGO
VS
DIZZINESS

WHAT IS THE DIFFERENCE BETWEEN VERTIGO AND DIZZINESS?

Meniere's is commonly described as a syndrome combining vertigo, fluctuating low frequency hearing loss, tinnitus and an aural pressure sensation. The symptoms may not necessarily occur simultaneously.

Meniere's causes severe disabling and unpredictable vertigo. The sudden episodes of vertigo arrive spontaneously. But what exactly is the difference between dizziness and Meniere's vertigo? Is vertigo just a more intensive form of dizziness? All vertigo comes with dizziness, but not all dizziness comes with vertigo. In most cases of dizziness, dizziness is not vertigo.

Vertigo is a lot different to feeling light headed and dizzy. Vertigo is an overwhelming sensation that the room is spinning around you. So even though you are lying or sitting still, the room feels to you, like it is moving around your body at an incredible speed. But of course it's an illusion. The room is the room; but vertigo creates an alarming shift. For you, the whole room is spinning. And it becomes much worse when you move your head even a millimetre. Your brain is in alarm mode and with a little extra movement it now receives extra signals that you are moving as well and this complicates the already mixed signals it's getting.

This massive equilibrium problem makes you vomit and become temporarily incapacitated. If someone walks into the room while you are 'spinning out' they will have no understanding of the inner spin you are involved with. They don't see or experience anything different. It's hard for anyone to contemplate what you are feeling right at that moment. You are alone in your distressing nightmare state of being. It is this dynamic illusion of movement that makes vertigo different from plain dizzy or common dizziness.

WHAT MAKES YOU HAVE A VERTIGO ATTACK?

In order to better understand Meniere's disease and vertigo, it is important to have a basic knowledge of the structure and function of the inner ear.

Inside the inner ear are two chambers called the scalae media and scalae vestibule. Only the scalae media contains endolymph, (potassium) while the scalae vestibule only contains perilymph (sodium). The scalae media and the scalae vestibule are separated by a membrane called the reissner's membrane.

The reissner membrane's primary function is to act as a diffusion barrier, allowing nutrients to travel from the perilymph to the endolymph chambers. No one knows for sure what happens. Although the general thinking is that fluid pressure builds up and stretches the reissner membrane that divides the two scalae compartments. As the membrane stretches, the symptoms of a vertigo attack start to happen.

It's in this 'beginning' of an oncoming attack that you'll experience your hearing and tinnitus getting worse. But the worst is yet to come. As the membrane becomes severely stretched, the fluids of the inner ear rupture the reissner. This results in the mixing of the scalae fluids, one rich in sodium, and the other rich in potassium. These fluids mix and flood the vestibular. It's this mixing and flooding that brings on the vertigo. After the membrane ruptures, it immediately starts to repair and heal. That's when you feel the vertigo diminishing.

HOW LONG DOES A VERTIGO ATTACK LAST?

Vertigo attacks are the most relentless and violent in the early stages of Meniere's disease. Vertigo attacks come at you with a vengeance. The unpredictable nature of the attacks, make the unknown duration and intensity of each episode even more frightening. But once a vertigo attack starts, it's anyone's guess how long the particular episode will last. Acutely distressing bouts of vertigo can last thirty minutes to hours. At other times, you may have signals that a vertigo attack is about to happen…but it doesn't. At other times you may feel woozy for weeks between major vertigo attacks. Other times, you may experience one vertigo attack after another. Or go for days, week, even months without having a vertigo attack.

THERE ARE THREE STAGES TO A VERTIGO ATTACK

THE BEGINNING.
THE MIDDLE.
THE END.

"After I discovered how to manage The Beginning, The Middle and The End stages effectively, I never suffered another vertigo attack."

-Meniere Man

An end to vertigo attacks does not happen overnight; you need to be consistent and committed to your own self-help management. So let's start at the beginning.

Most things in nature have recognizable patterns. The mind finds it easier to accept patterns, rather than randomness. Something with a pattern becomes familiar. And understandable, like a trip to the mountain, a birth of a new baby, or green leaves emerging in Spring. When we recognise patterns we lose the chaos and start to find understanding.

The recognition that vertigo attacks have a pattern, was a major step forward physically and psychologically for me. While vertigo is not something you look forward to, it does have a pattern you can recognize.

I call the three stages of Meniere's vertigo, the B.M.E. Each vertigo attack has a Beginning, Middle and End. When you know this B.M.E. pattern, you can use self-help techniques to gain control during each of the three stages of a vertigo attack. Then you'll see symptoms as sign posts on your path to a full recovery.

THE BEGINNING

HOW TO HELP YOURSELF IN THE BEGINNING

FIRST RECOGNIZE THE FIVE SYMPTOMS OF THE BEGINNING STAGE

1. Increased tinnitus/loud, roaring, screeching sounds.

2. Aural fullness/fullness feeling of pressure in your ear.

3. Increased tiredness or yawning for no apparent reason.

4. Feeling off-balance.

5. Decreased hearing.

Any of these symptoms can indicate the beginning stage of a vertigo attack. Inside your inner ear the reissner membrane is already being stretched and fluid is building up in your vestibular. All of these symptoms may happen over a day or two.

The sooner you recognise this beginning stage the better. If you take action, you have more opportunity of avoiding the attack. Or lessening the intensity. Whatever you do, take this beginning stage seriously. Take control and help yourself. If you are experiencing the beginning symptoms of a Meniere's vertigo attack, you need to put measures in place for a day or two. I'm serious. This is the time to pay attention to your body.

I found that by treating the beginning stage seriously, attacks would often *not* develop. I used these techniques regularly, until the intensity of my attacks became less; the time between attacks became longer and eventually I managed to avoid vertigo attacks altogether. Which is exactly what you want to get to. So be consistent and committed to your own self-help management. It is not difficult and it feels great to look after yourself.

Here is how it works. When any of the five warning symptoms appear, STOP doing what you're doing immediately! And do the following.

1. Pay attention to how you move. Make your movements controlled and fluid .

2. Avoid sudden movements with your head, eyes or body.

3. Avoid tipping your head back to look up.

4. If you need to bend down to pick up things, do this action slowly.

5. If you feel dizzy or woozy, simply sit or lie in one position until the feeling passes, can be half an hour.

6. Avoid excessive electronic gadget use: internet, smartphone, laptop, iPad.

7. Don't watch television, videos, movies or work on the computer. Avoid constant exposure to artificial light. Rest your eyes. Remember the eyes, are directly connected to your vestibular system.

8. Don't drive or go in a moving vehicle. Rest your balance and vestibular system by not making demands on it.

9. Avoid caffeine. You must find something palatable to substitute for caffeine. Certain teas like chamomile, raspberry, rose hip or peppermint are soothing and have health giving properties.

10. Don't drink alcohol.

11. Don't smoke.

12. Avoid sugar: artificial drinks, energy drinks and amphetamine variants, and all refined sugars. No artificial sweeteners.

13. Make a lemon and honey drink. Lemon helps vertigo symptoms.

14. Drink ginger tea. The properties in ginger root are known to help vertigo symptoms. Make your own tea by mixing 1 teaspoon fresh grated ginger root and 1 teaspoon honey in a cup of boiling water. Strain.

15. Eat small protein-rich meals. Over eating stresses your body. Avoid simple carbohydrates like white flour products (cakes, breads, puddings).

16. Avoid all salt, nitrates, sodium enriched foods, processed foods and preservatives.

17. Eat potassium rich bananas.

18. Take a bath. Water helps relaxation and stops the feeling of anxiety and panic. Add a few drops of aromatherapy essential oils into the bath. Symptomatic treatment through aromatherapy (using genuine pure essential oils only) act to sooth the nerves. Try orange blossom, geranium,

ylang ylang, jasmine, lavender or rose oil.

19. Also use aromatherapy oils in an oil burner or room vaporizer. Helps calm and regulate thoughts, affects wellbeing and has a restorative function.

20. Listen to a meditation cd or soothing music.

21. Get someone to re-schedule business and social commitments.

22. Don't try to think or figure anything out. Stay away from all mental and emotional stress.

23. No late-nights and early morning schedules. Go to bed early. Sleep has a restorative function.

24. Get a quality nights sleep. Don't use the computer before sleep as it keeps your brain awake.

25. Tell people how you are feeling! Ask them to help you out with anything you need.

Take note that relaxation and cessation of normal activities is not just for half an hour. It's for as long as it takes until symptoms go away.

To work towards being vertigo free, you need to apply these strategies.

THE MIDDLE

HOW TO HELP YOURSELF IN THE MIDDLE STAGE.

COPING TECHNIQUES FOR THE MIDDLE STAGE OF THE ROTATIONAL VERTIGO ATTACK

The middle stage is the most dynamic stage of the vertigo attack. You may have a few minutes to realize that there is no going back. You'll definitely be experiencing serious dizziness which is quickly developing into nystagmus, where your eyes feel like they're following the room moving around you. This may take place over three to four minutes, but you are still mobile enough to find a place to lie down. After that, you are into a rotational spinning vertigo attack. This lasts for at least thirty minutes to an hour.

Towards the end of the attack you will notice the spinning is a little less severe. As the spinning slows down, you are managing to see something specific in the room, before it spins away. Slowly you are able to focus on a window or a picture. Once focusing on an object becomes possible, you start feeling you can get control back. Finally, there won't be any more spinning and you'll be able to sleep.

GET TO A SAFE SETTING

When the attack begins, lie down in a safe place. This sounds obvious, but unless you do, you could find yourself in physical danger or social difficulty.

PHARMACY RESCUE

There are various anti-vertigo drugs available that can make you feel better during the initial or severe phases of vertigo. Vestibular sedatives generally mask the vertigo by decreasing the brain's response to vestibular input. These drugs are Antivert, Droperidol, Compazine, Valium, Ativan. Talk to your doctor about these and other drug options.

GET COMFORTABLE

Make yourself as comfortable as possible. Dim the lights or draw the blinds. Avoid noise. A quiet room helps you relax more. The more you can relax, the less severe your symptoms will be. And the sooner you will recover your equilibrium.

DONT LIE FLAT

Don't lie down flat. This increases the sense of disorientation. Use two pillows, or something that elevates your head.

KEEP YOUR EYES OPEN

Don't shut your eyes completely. Leave them slightly open. Don't use your eyes to keep track of the furniture moving around the room or attempt to stop the spinning. You will only feel worse and become more anxious.

AVOID MOVEMENT

The vestibular nerve is already challenged with the attack. So any other demands only intensify the sense of spinning. You may have to move your head or shift your body position. If you change position, move *very, very slowly.*

RELAX AND BREATHE

If you tense your body, shallow-breathe or hold your breath, it makes the vertigo attack seem worse. But if you relax your body and breathe slowly and deeply, you get more oxygen into your body and the panic reaction reduces. So try to breathe deeply.

Try to "soften" the attack relaxe your body. Is your breath high in your chest? If it is, drop your breathing down to your belly. Even this one relaxation technique will help you. Pay attention to how you're breathing rather than focusing on the spinning.

MIND CONTROL

As you are experiencing the vertigo attack, you can think; the cycle has begun; now you are moving forwards towards the end of the vertigo attack. You can't go back and prevent it happening, but you know and accept the attack will end.

Negative self talk increases anxiety. The more you minimize anxiety, the less the cycle of anxiety and fear will carry you away and intensify an attack. Remind yourself that you will not be trapped in this experience forever. Although it may feel like it at the time. Negative thoughts of how awful it is, or how you can't stand it, how bad it is and so on, fuel panic thoughts and fear.

Your mind is something that you can

control. So interrupt negative thoughts you're having. I don't want to sound glib here, but if you don't mentally fight against it, the spinning seems less intense. The less shock you have, the quicker your body will naturally repair. So the most effective coping tool you have at this stage is your mind. Mind over matter works well for vertigo attacks.

7 POWERFUL SENTENCES TO PUT YOU IN CONTROL DURING THE MIDDLE STAGE OF A ROTATIONAL VERTIGO ATTACK

Chose one or two sentences that resonate with you or make up similar ones. Write these out in advance and make a phrase that you can easily remember when you are having an attack of vertigo.

1. I am O.K.
2. This will pass soon.
3. I'm safe.
4. My inner ear will heal itself.
5. This won't last forever.
6. Feel calm.
7. Go with it.

KEEP THIS IN MIND:

- Accept the vertigo experiencing.

- Don't fight against the vertigo attack.

- Remind yourself that the vertigo attack is only temporary and it will pass.

- Self talk the vertigo attack down in importance.

- Remind yourself that you are not in any danger.

- Change negative self talk into positive self talk.

- Realize that when the vertigo sensations feel at the worst point, you'll soon recover.

THE END

HOW TO HELP YOURSELF AT THE END STAGE

FOCUS ON A FIXED POINT

As the spinning subsides a little try to find a focus on something, just above eye level directly in front of you. A picture, a spot on the wall, or a door handle. Whatever is in front of you. You won't be able to focus this way, until the attack lessens. But do it as soon as you can. If the spot slides away slowly bring your focus back to the point. Repeat this until it is possible to stay focused on that point. At this stage you know that the reissner is healing and you will soon be in the stage of recovery.

Learn to listen to your body. If you have suffered a severe vertigo episode that has left you exhausted, then common sense tells you to rest or sleep before you attempt to get up. Remember you are in a recovery mode and need to replenish your body. An attack is a serious physiological trauma.

The end stage is about recovery. Emotionally you feel a great sense of relief. During this final stage, the vertigo has stopped and you have slept or rested for a couple of hours. You won't be able to concentrate or do physically demanding activities. You'll be feeling very tired and will need to rest regularly. The feeling in this stage is one of vulnerability. Not dizzy but not anchored either. I call it woozy. So you can't be physically decisive at this stage. Balance is not fully restored. But you're pleased to be back in the land of gravity once again. The only things still moving are the hands on the clock.

It takes time to gain a sense of full recovery from an attack. I found after the attack I was in a recovery mode for a few days. I often tried to shorten this stage down to a couple of hours so I could get back to normal. But this stage is an important biological healing time. If you try to push through this end stage you may undo the healing that is taking place and have another attack.

After a year of attacks, I worked out the end stage can be three days to a week. This is a very valuable time for healing. And you must take advantage to heal well. It does take time. Here are my suggestions to get you back on your feet and feeling normal.

VISUALIZATION EXERCISE TO DO ONCE YOU ARE ABLE TO FOCUS ON A FIXED POINT

The practise of positive visualization and positive thinking in helping manage physical symptoms was well-documented by Emil Coué, in the early 1900's. He asserted that all of your thoughts become reality. The power of imagination is greater than the power of the will. You are what you think. If you think unhappy thoughts, you become sad.

So taking Emil Coué's approach that the mind is a powerful healing tool, you can use your mind to help overcome the intense fear you feel during an attack. Instead of tensing up and letting the worse happen...you can refocus your mind on positive healing images instead.

Visualization is a form of energy. It is effective in helping with the specific anxiety and stress that vertigo attacks cause.

Creating a positive healing image is easy to do. One of the best scenarios I had in my mind was the following. First, I'd visualize the inner ear structure, especially the reissner membrane and scalae fluids. I'd imagine the reissner membrane repairing. Then the fluids passing naturally through the reissner. I'd imagine an even flow of white light flowing through my inner ear. Next, my inner ear slowly returning to a natural, stable balanced state. I'd repeat this visualization during the later stages of the attack, until I felt comfortable. Each time, I told myself I was healing and getting stronger and that balance was a natural state.

Everything is energy and our minds through visualization help create our recovery. Don't wait passively for the Meniere attack to be completely over. Do this as soon as you can.

VISUALIZATIION EXCERCISE

1. Imagine you see the reissner membrane.

2. See the reissner membrane healing.

3. All the healing fluids are passing naturally through the reissner.

4. Now there is an even flow of life fluids moving in your inner ear.

5. Say to yourself... my inner ear is slowly returning to its natural balance.

6. Balance is a natural state of being.

7. See yourself healing, getting stronger and in prefect balance.

DURING THE END STAGE TRY THIS SIMPLE FIVE FINGER EXERCISE TO RELAX

Do the finger exercises below and in less than ten minutes you can feel a greater sense of inner peace.

Breathe slowly and deeply.

1. Touch your thumb to your index finger. Think of a time in the past when your body felt very warm and relaxed, such as laying in a hammock, sitting in the sand on a warm day, or after swimming, jogging, walking, skiing or playing tennis. Relax and enjoy the feeling for a while.

2. Touch your thumb to your middle finger. Think of a time in the past when you had a truly loving experience, an intimate conversation, a hug, stroking a pet. Remember how good the feeling

was. Hold that feeling for a while.

3. Touch your thumb to your ring finger. Think of the time in the past when someone gave you a compliment. Think of the conversation and what you said. Imagine paying them a compliment back.

4. Touch your thumb to your little finger. Think of a beautiful place you have been to. Look around. See the most beautiful place in detail. Stay in that place for a while.

DRINK

Drink water. Hydrate yourself to counter the effects of body shock. Stay hydrated after a vertigo attack. Drink pure mineral water with high levels of magnesium and low sodium content. Avoid caffeine. Or caffeinated drinks. Caffeine increases dehydration. And that's not what you need at this stage.

Small actions go a long way to recovery. Try making a cup of ginger tea. This can be made by washing and peeling fresh ginger root and grating it into a teapot. One tablespoon of grated ginger makes about four cups. Pour boiling water over. Seep for 5 minutes. Sweeten with a teaspoon or two of unprocessed natural honey. Sip slowly. Drink hot or cold.

A word of warning though. Do not take ginger if you have a bile duct obstruction or gallstones. Ginger may stimulate bile production. High doses of ginger (6 grams or more) can cause damage to the stomach lining and ulcers. Ginger can cause allergic skin reactions. Consult your doctor before taking ginger if you take blood thinners.

Also green tea is a natural source of anti-oxidants. Or a large glass of freshly squeezed orange juice. Drink the juice slowly chewing each mouthful so the vitamin C is absorbed through the mucus membranes in your mouth.

EAT

Eat a banana. Potassium rich, and with natural sugars, a banana gives your body a much needed boost of vitamins, minerals and energy to get you back on your feet quickly.

Bananas give you a quick natural pick up

of blood sugar levels. Eat poppy seeds or a few almonds, raisins, figs, apricots, or cranberries (preferably organic, without preservatives).

WATER

Take a long hot bath with essential oils to relax your nerves. Or a hot shower. Let the water run over the back of your neck and down your spine. Breathe and relax. Shake your hands as you let go the vertigo experience. The properties of water remove negative ions from your body. This will refresh and relax you.

AROMATHERAPY OILS

A few small bottles of 100% pure essential is a great investment. A few drops is all you need to calm tensions, relieve stress and help promote restful and repairing sleep. Relaxing lavender, soothing ylang ylang or rose, balancing geranium, or naturally tranquilizing mandarin orange.

Place 5-10 drops of oil with warm water into an oil burner for essential oils. Add a few drops of your choice into a warm bath.

Mix two drops with a carrier oil such as

almond oil for a self massage of your feet. Or have someone who cares for your well-being; give you a gentle whole body massage, especially your feet, hands, shoulders and back.

CONNECT

Stand outdoors. Look at the horizon. Breathe. Listen and look at nature. This will help reconnect you to the world.

HELPING HANDS

You can use your hands to simply apply physical pressure to help you connect to your body and gain a sense of balance again.

Cup your hands over your eyes for five seconds while you breathe deeply. The warmth and darkness are comforting.

Half close your eyes; place your right hand across your forehead. Doing this helps your head orient with the rest of your body. Press your forehead against your hand.

Place a hand on each side of your head above your ear. Perform the counter-pressure exercise on each side.

Place your fingertips on your forehead.

Press your forehead against your fingertips. Try to keep your fingers from being pushed back by your head.

MOVE

Get up and moving as soon as you can. Moving assists your brain to compensate for the imbalance. Correct adjustment to vestibular imbalance, is a process known as compensation. Vestibular compensation is a process that allows the brain to regain balance control and minimize dizziness symptoms.

When you have an imbalance between the right and left vestibular organs, the key component to successful adaptation is a dedicated effort to keep moving. By moving and doing things, (despite still feeling 'woozy') you strengthen the balance system. As you move, you're helping your body and brain regain the ability to process balance information. Remember this is at the End stage of the B.M.E. The objective here is to go slowly but definitely get going.

DO

Do things you like to do. Spend time with family and friends. Walk. Eat out. Shop. Don't let the vertigo attack you've just had, keep you at home. It's over. Move about. Move on. Have fun.

Learn to listen to your body. If you have suffered a severe vertigo episode that has left you exhausted, then common sense tells you to rest or sleep before you attempt to get up. Remember you are in a recovery mode and need to replenish your body. An attack is a serious physiological trauma.

The end stage is about recovery. Emotionally you feel a great sense of relief. During this final stage, the vertigo has stopped and you have slept or rested for a couple of hours. You won't be able to concentrate or do physically demanding activities. You'll be feeling very tired and will need to rest regularly. The feeling in this stage is one of vulnerability. Not dizzy but not anchored either. I call it woozy. So you can't be physically decisive at this stage. Balance is not fully restored. But you're pleased to be back in the land of gravity once again. The only things still moving are the hands on the clock.

It takes time to gain a sense of full recovery from an attack. I found after the attack I was in a recovery mode for a few days. I often tried to shorten this stage down to a couple of hours so I could get back to normal. But this stage is an important biological healing time. If you try to push through this end stage you may undo the healing that is taking place and have another attack.

After a year of attacks, I worked out the end stage can be three days to a week. This is a very valuable time for healing. And you must take advantage to heal well. It does take time.

The explanations and managment of the BME (three stages) will help, get you back on your feet and feeling normal.

It does work.

Stay positive and hopeful.

ANTI-VERTIGO NOTEBOOK

In contrast to seeing Meniere's as purely anxious and stressful, try to see Meniere's as a life challenge. Make a definite choice to take control of your circumstances. Make a commitment to yourself that you will do all you can to support your physical and mental well-being.

Taking control of your situation is not a magic wand and instant fix, but it does create a personal focus on wellness.

This focus is helped enormously by keeping a notebook of daily activities and how that affected your ymptoms.

If you take a close look at how you are living your life, you can make significant changes that will ultimately improve your health and help you manage vertigo symptoms. This in turn will improve your health status and bring about a balance in your new world.

By making notes on how you are feeling after and during your day to day activities you will see a pattern emerging. Some will be bad and some will be good. With notes you can clearly establish what activities are aggravating or helping your situation.

Remember bad feelings must be eliminated. How you do things is a personal revelation. No one can say for sure what changes you need to make. It's something you must figure for yourself.

When you think about it, you can put so many good and healthy measures in place. Relaxation, mind control, exercise and diet to cope with Meniere's disease. Your focus will change from a disastrous Meniere life to a healthy powerful one.

Your health is up to you.

40 WAYS TO HELP YOURSELF GET OVER MENIERE'S VERTIGO

1. Learn and practise deep breathing excersises.

2. Eat a heathy low salt diet.

3. Practise stress reducing techniques.

4. Take time to relax, breathe and unwind at least twice a day.

5. Maintain a nutritional salt-reduced diet.

6. Nurture and support your own needs.

7. Work smarter, not harder.

8. Avoid alcohol.

9. Avoid smoking and second-hand cigarette smoke.

10. Take personal time out just for yourself.

11. Get enough sleep each night.

12. Take a power nap of 20-30 minutes each day.

13. Use humor to nurture an attitude of happiness.

14. Spend time with friends and family.

15. Work smarter not harder.

16. Identify your personal interests and keep involved in doing what you love to do.

17. Learn meditation and practise everyday.

18. Focus on what you can control.

19. Avoid peer pressure.

20. Walk away from stress.

21. Avoid work-related stress.

22. Avoid arguments.

23. Avoid a constant fast-paced lifestyle.

24. Avoid excessive use of electronic gadgets.

25. Avoid constant exposure to artificial light.

26. Manage social obligations to suit yourself rather than letting them manage you.

27. Make each day have a purpose. Even a single purpose is enough. Avoid purposeless days.

28. Avoid addictions to late-night serials on television. Get quality sleep.

29. Take regular breaks when using the internet and computers.

30. Avoid recreational drugs.

31. Remember that lifestyle and diet are vital to your recovery.

32. Look at stresses you are under and your workload.And do something about them.

33. Exercise regularly. Walk everyday if possible.

34. Practice setting goals.

35. Create a daily routine.

36. Don't rush. Pace yourself. Things will get done in their own time

37. Be patient with yourself.

38. Focus on one or two essential tasks a day. Prioritize, you don't have to complete everything in one day.

39. Be kind and have compassion and empathy for yourself.

40. Be your own best friend.

12 HEALTHY EATING GUIDELINES FOR VERTIGO SUFFERERS

I'm not exactly a health food nut, as the term goes, but I do appreciate the taste of real food: raw, fresh, unprocessed and organic. By eating real and healthy foods, you are working towards a vertigo free life.

You can affect your body in the future by the choices you make today.

Here are twelve of my tried and tested

eating guidelines that will point your shopping cart in the right direction.

SALTY TALK

Sodium creates an imbalance in the body's fluids, especially in the inner ear. This can trigger vertigo. So one goal for managing Meniere's vertigo, is to reduce the total body fluid volume. According to the University of Maryland Medical Centre, treatment for Meniere's disease is directed towards attempts to decrease the fluid pressure in the inner ear by avoiding substances that may trigger or exacerbate fluid pressure build up in the inner ear.

According to the University of Maryland Medical Centre, maintaining a low-salt diet involves restricting sodium intake to between 1,500 to 2,000 milligrams per day. Sodium causes fluid retention, so you will need to reduce your salt intake. I reduced my salt intact to 1000-1500 mg a day. We are not talking a total no salt diet. Don't try to eliminate salt altogether; your muscles and nerves need it to function.

The average western diet consumes just over 3,000 milligrams of sodium each day. You can't live without salt, but you don't need as much salt to live! Remember the goal is to reduce your daily sodium intake to 1000-2000 milligrams. This involves more than not sprinkling salt on your food. It requires diligence in precisely measuring your sodium intake from all sources by inspecting package labels and kitchen habits.

When planning a low salt diet, you can read books on low-salt diets or consult a nutritionist to establish a salt-restricted diet and help keep track of your sodium intake. Cutting down on salt is one good thing, but if you eat enough foods rich in potassium, you may not have to cut back so much on the salt. That's where a registered dietician can help you with a specific diet plan tailored for you.

Maintain a low salt intake on a daily basis. Avoid adding salt to food while cooking. Don't add salt to meals at the table. Throw away the salt shaker. It doesn't make sense to not put salt into the dish you're cooking but shake it over your plate at the table. Salting your food is not an option. Adding salt may be the first habit you give up.

One of the best ways to change a habit is to not buy any salt or salted foods or bring them into the house. Let your family know why they need to read labels too. Whoever is cooking dinner, needs to look at how much salt goes into the recipes and modify. That's how friends and family can get involved rather than inadvertently sabotaging or compromising your aim at reducing salt down.

Most sodium comes in the familiar form of table salt. But other chemical compounds also contain sodium. Even diet drinks, such as diet soda, contain sodium. Some brands of bottled water can have high sodium content especially if carbonated. Just a few changes to food and beverage choices makes a difference to lowering your daily total of sodium.

PROCESSED FOODS

A general low-salt rule, avoid or limit processed foods that are high in sodium, canned vegetables and soups, spaghetti sauce, vegetable juices and ready-to-eat cereals. Avoid high salt foods like ravioli, salted nuts, potato crisps, broth, bouillon cubes and gravies.

Delicious as they are, ham, sausage, bacon, liver, offal are also offenders in salt overload. So avoid smoked, cured, salted and canned meats.

Read labels and avoid sodium saccharin

(a sugar substitute), disodium phosphate (a preservative), monosodium glutamate and trisodium phosphate.

CHEESE

Your only use for hard cheese should be in a mousetrap. This is the end of the cheese board as you know it. Say goodbye to aged cheddar, and blue vein. Gorgonzola is out. Avoid soft cheeses including cheese sauces, cheese spreads, processed cheese, processed cheese, and cheese dips.

BAKEHOUSE BLUES

The more processed a grain is, the more likely it is to be high in sodium. This list is more than a baker's dozen. Breads and rolls, quick breads, self-rising flour, pancake mix, pizza, biscuits, bread crumb coatings, croutons, salted crackers and pretzels.

VEGE VILLIANS

Avoid canned and packet vegetable juices, olives, dill pickles, sauerkraut, pickled vegetables and relishes, pasta and tomato sauces, bottled salad dressings, regular peanut butter, soy sauce and sauces like BBQ seasonings, rubs and marinades. Make your own at home and leave the salt out.

LOW SALT SHOPPING

Many choices of low salt foods are available in supermarkets, food stores and markets. It's easy to replace high salt foods with low-salt foods. Here's an example. Instead of crackers with a high salt content, choose a brand with the lowest salt content. You can still eat foods you love, you just have to change the brands and put low salt packets, cans or cartons into your shopping trolley.

We've talked about foods you should avoid. Here's a list of foods you can eat: Low-fat dairy products such as low-salt cheese, lean organic meat, water-packed tuna, fresh or frozen vegetables, fresh or frozen fruits, whole grain bread, low-salt biscuits and crackers. Whole grain cereals such as oats, enriched cereals like Grapenuts, unsalted popcorn, fresh salads, bottled or packet low-sodium salad dressings.

AVOID FAST FOOD

To help promote blood viscosity and improve blood supply to the inner ear and brain, it's important to reduce the amount of saturated fats and trans fats you eat. These types of fats are commonly found in meats, oils, fast foods and processed foods.

Cholesterol is a waxy substance that travels through the bloodstream to all the body's cells. While cholesterol has important functions in the body, excessive amounts of cholesterol may adversely affect circulation of blood to the inner ear.

You can control cholesterol levels in the body by controlling the amount of high cholesterol foods you eat. The first step is to throw the deep fryer away. Avoid all fried foods, (especially deep-fried foods) and grill, bake, poach, instead of frying.

The second step to reducing cholesterol, is to reduce your intake of ice cream, cheese, milk, mayonnaise, butter and meat.

The Mayo Clinic also published a list of the top five foods that can help lower cholesterol levels in the body. Their list of cholesterol reducing foods include: high soluble fiber foods like oatmeal, apples, pears, prunes and kidney beans; walnuts and almonds; foods high in omega-3 fatty acids are tuna, salmon, sardines, canola oil, and olive oil.

THE UNLOVING SPOONFUL

If you love a teaspoon of sugar in your tea, you need to give it up. Sugars raise blood pressure and blood sugar temporarily. When your blood sugar is high, the blood takes longer to circulate to reach your brain.

Simple sugars are 'bad' sugars. Because almost as soon as you eat them, they cause a sudden spike, (sugar high) followed by a sudden drop in blood sugar levels. This sudden spike and drop is thought to be a possible trigger for a Meniere's vertigo attack.

To lower the level of blood sugar in your body, it is important to cut out simple carbohydrates and simple sugars from your diet. Instead, go for complex carbohydrates, which are known to stabilize the body's blood sugar levels.

The following foods should be reduced or eliminated from your diet: concentrated fruit juice, candy, cookies, biscuits, cakes, muffins, donuts, sweets, pastas and breads made with white flour, sugary cereals, white sugar, ice cream, milk chocolate (go for dark chocolate). No jams. No soda drinks.

THE SOURCE OF GOOD CARBS

The opposite of the simple sugar spike, is the slow burning energy of complex carbohydrates. When you replace foods with simple sugars for more complex carbohydrates, you feel the benefits of no sugar rushes and you'll find you're less exhausted.

Whole grain bread, brown rice, legumes like dried beans, pulses and lentils, vegetables, barley, wild rice, soy beans, fruits, nuts and seeds. All of these complex carbohydrates have multiple benefits such as reducing cholesterol and giving you more energy. Not only do they taste great, they're a great way to get minerals and vitamins your body needs to heal.

THE SUPER SUPPLEMENT

You don't need much salt to live a healthy life, but if your salt level is under the recommended level for a healthy body, that can be a health hazard. So you have to get the balance right. You need some salt and you also need potassium for health.

Potassium is a major positive ion inside human cells and helps cells with body functions. Contracting your muscles requires potassium. From lifting your eyebrow, to lifting a finger. Your heart is a muscle that contracts too. So get potassium for heart function and also brain function.

Potassium has been linked to the prevention of major medical conditions. Potassium is the great 'reducer'. This mineral helps lower blood pressure; reduce the risk of stroke, reduce the risk of heart disease, reduce the chances of developing kidney stones, and amazingly, potassium reduces the body's sensitivity to salt. This reduction of sensitivity is a good reason for Meniere's sufferers to ask the doctor for a potassium sparing diuretic.

As well as taking a potassium sparing diuretic, you can counteract potassium depletion naturally, by increasing your potassium in your daily diet. Most people consume only about half of the daily recommended amount of potassium.

ALL THE FOLLOWING FOODS CONTAIN HIGH LEVELS OF POTASSIUM

So what foods contain generous helpings of potassium? One abundant source of potassium is avocado. A whole avocado contains around 1,100 mg. A great reason to make guacamole.

Fruits contain large amounts of potassium. The richest sources are bananas, one medium banana has 422 mg. Half cup of fresh plums provides a 530 mg of potassium. A half cup of dried raisins contains nearly 600 mg of potassium. One medium orange, 237 mg. A medium potato baked with skin on provides 926 mg of potassium. Cantaloupe melon, apricots, orange juice, sweet potatoes, green beans, broccoli, green peppers, asparagus, turnips, parsnips, tomatoes, soybeans, brown rice and garlic. Cocoa and chocolate are high potassium: An ounce of chocolate has about 120 mg of potassium.

Almonds 200 mg. Brazil nuts 170 mg. Sunflower seeds 200 mg of potassium.

Instead of salt for taste, use herbs and spices to replace salt in cooking. These add flavour and taste to dishes. Some herbs and spices contain potassium. One tablespoon of parsley gives you 16 mg of potassium. So if you make Middle Eastern salad with a cup of chopped parsley, and four cloves of garlic (at 12 mg of potassium each), now you're cooking. One teaspoon of dill seeds 25 mg. Other sources of potassium are celery and cress. Once you understand food values, it's easy to cook without salt while increasing your potassium intake.

BREATHING WILL HELP YOU WITH VERTIGO ATTACKS AND INCREASE YOUR OVERALL HEALTH AND VITALITY

Breathing is life. When your breathing is poor, inflow of oxygen is less and the flow of waste gases from the body is reduced. This makes it harder to cope with a stressful vertigo attack. In fact, poor breathing exasperate the vertigo experience causing more panic, more anxiety and exhaustion.

However, when you practise breathing awareness and good breathing techniques, you can use your breath for first aid during a vertigo attack. You can learn to use your breathing to calm yourself.

There are two ways of breathing. Shallow chest breathing or deep abdominal breathing. When you are feeling anxious or suffering stress in your life, your breathing is chest breathing, shallow, irregular and often fast. Less air enters the lungs; heart rate, muscle tension and stress levels increase.

Breathing from your diaphragm (deep abdominal breathing) is the natural way to reduce stress levels. This is the natural way the body breathes. It's what we do in our sleep or when we are unconscious. Air is inhaled deep into the lungs and completely exhaled. Energy gained from the oxygen, helps you relax. But when we are conscious we tend to breathe only from the chest and consequently make half breaths.

Practising good breathing techniques is the easiest way to gain a sense of relaxation and stress release. Abdominal breathing exercises will reduce anxiety and oxygenate your cells. When your cells have oxygen, the body has a greater chance of returning to a healthy state quickly. You will also experience a better sense of wellbeing. Less anxiety, less panicky, less depression, less irritability, reduced muscle tension and less tiredness.

It takes a little practise to breathe through your belly and then into your chest. Persistent practise will help you feel better day by day.

Breathing techniques can be learned in no time and the benefits felt immediately. But long-term effects of breathing won't be noticed until you have spent a few months of everyday practise.

THE ABDOMINAL BREATHING TECHNIQUE

To breathe deeply, begin by putting your hand on your abdomen just below the navel.

Close your eyes.

Breathe in, as if you are breathing in through your belly.

Make your belly fill with air and feel it expand.

Move the breath up into your chest and feel it expand.

Hold the breath for a few seconds, exhale slowly.

Inhale again slowly through your nose, feel your hand move out as your belly expands.

Move the same breath up and expand your chest.

Now exhale, make sure you expel all your breath by pulling in your diaphragm and expelling all the air from your lower lungs. Repeat.

VESTIBULAR REHABILITATION TO GET YOU BALANCED

If you experience problems with your balance between episodes of vertigo, you may benefit from vestibular rehabilitation therapy to help the development of vestibular compensation. Then you'll be up and about doing the things you want to be doing. Vestibular exercises were not around when I was diagnosed with Meniere's disease, but I have included this updated information in this edition.

No one told me about vestibular rehabilitation, because no one knew. But left to my own to figure this, I went on my 'gut' feeling and decided to do more balance activities to make my vestibular system work harder and improve my balance.

The list is a long one during the Meniere years. I walked until I was able to jog; learned to windsurf, water skied, learned to ski, learned to do weight training, learned how to stretch and do core balance workouts on the Swiss ball, cycled, snow boarded, swam in the pool, swam in the ocean, surfed again, climbed ladders, gardened, pruned trees, read books, went sailing, went fishing, snorkelled, travelled by air, by car etc! Phew! I did all of this between attacks of vertigo.

Sometimes during an active weekend, I'd have a vertigo attack. No wonder! My balance system was doing a full range of compensating tasks. Yes I had an attack but I was not only developing my vestibular ability I spent normal family time plus I was still doing life. So it wasn't all bad.

Everything you do helps, whether you snow ski, throw a tennis ball to the dog or plant bulbs in the garden. Every movement incorporates body balance. That's why, when you do things, you can sometimes feel bad. But if you accept dizziness or vertigo as a necessary part of the healing process, fear of doing things won't come into the equation.

When you see dizziness and even a vertigo attack as a sign that an imbalance in your vestibular systems still exists, you need to believe that every physical activity you do, is helping you recover your life. It is like tough love for vertigo. Laying around in bed doesn't help you get anywhere. But getting up and having a go, goes a long way, towards getting a full and active life back again.

See every movement of exercise, whether it is with a physiotherapist or something you enjoy doing on your own (like gardening, cooking or some sport) as strengthening your vestibular ability. Do what you love to do. If you experience problems with your balance between episodes of vertigo, you may benefit from vestibular rehabilitation therapy. The goal of V.R.T. (Vestibular Rehabilitation Therapy) is to retrain the brain to recognise and process signals from the vestibular system in co-ordination with information from vision and body.

Essentially, the brain copes with the disorienting signals coming from the inner ear by learning to rely more on the alternative signals coming from the eyes, ankles, legs, spine, neck and muscular system to maintain balance. Vestibular compensation can even be successfully achieved when the damage to the inner ear is permanent.

A qualified therapist will first give you a thorough evaluation. This includes observing your posture, balance, movement, and compensatory strategies you're already doing. Using the result of this evaluation, the therapist will develop an individual treatment plan designed to include exercises that combine specific head and body movements with eye exercises and activities that you perform during therapy sessions and also do at home.

These exercises involve movements of the eyes, the head, the upper body, and then the whole body under different visual situations (for example, with the eyes open or closed, or looking at steady objects or a moving ball), on different surfaces and in different environments.

As you can guess, some of the exercises and activities may at first cause an increase in symptoms, as body and brain attempt to sort out the new pattern of movements. A key factor is that the brain must sense the presence of imbalance to begin the process of vestibular compensation. So with time and consistent work, the signals from the eyes, body and vestibular system will start to co-ordinate again. This gives a greater sense of balance. Which is just what you need.

Some physiotherapists use a set pattern of exercises known as the Cawthorn–Cooksey exercises, named after the two people responsible for devising them. The aims of the Cawthorn-Cooksey exercises include relaxing the neck and shoulder muscles, training the eyes to move independently of the head, practicing good balance in everyday situations, practicing the head movements that cause dizziness (to help the development of vestibular compensation), improving general co-ordination, and encouraging natural spontaneous movement.

You should be assessed for an individual exercise program to ensure you are doing the appropriate exercises for your specific issues. You will be given guidance on how many repetitions of each exercise to do and when to progress to the next set of exercises. Your doctor can refer you.

This is an example of the type of rehabilitation excercises from Cawthorne Cooksey

VESTIBULAR EXERCISES

IN BED OR SITTING

Eye movements -- at first slow, then quick

up and down

from side to side

Focusing on finger moving from 3 feet to 1 foot away from face

Head movements at first slow, then quick, later with eyes closed

bending forward and backward

turning from side to side.

SITTING

Eye movements and head movements as above

Shoulder shrugging and circling

Bending forward and picking up objects from the ground

STANDING

Eye, head and shoulder movements as before

Changing from sitting to standing position with eyes open and shut

Throwing a small ball from hand to hand (above eye level)

Throwing a ball from hand to hand under knee

Changing from sitting to standing and turning around in between.

THE STIGMA OF MENIERE'S

Vertigo is not just a physiological issue, it's also a psychological one. And this affects more than the moment of vertigo. It affects you on a daily basis. And it affects how you relate to others around you.

The psychologist Goffman (1963) says "An individual carries a stigma if she/he is unable for any reason to fulfil society's stereotypic criteria for normality - if this deviation is obvious (e.g. physical deformity) the person is at once 'discredited'. Failings that are less obvious or may be concealed (e.g. vestibular problems) render the individual 'discreditable' in the sense that his/her identity is vulnerable. Whereas a discredited person must adopt a stigmatized identity - a discreditable individual may prefer the effort and risks attached to trying to 'pass' as normal to the frank stigma of admitting the attribute". How is this for a learned evaluation of your inner condition of Meniere's disease?

I can relate to what Goffman is saying here. I was one of the people who tried to pass as normal at work. I "acted" normal, as if I did not have anything wrong with me and dodged showing any symptoms. I didn't wish to have the stigma of admitting the symptoms because I felt my identity was extremely vulnerable. This identity issue is something you are going to need specialized help for. You must come to terms with it in a positive productive manner.

Personally, I found that once I accepted that Meniere's was a permanent part of my life, I started to be able to work with and live with the symptoms. Once I could accept the symptoms, I became more aware of how they were presented to me. I became aware that there was a pattern to every vertigo attack. I made changes to my lifestyle and attitude. And so the acceptance of the condition became, by default, part of the healing process. I accepted that it was up to me to make changes and take charge.

QUALITY OF WELL-BEING AND YOU

If you think you felt bad, well the good news is you're right! It's not your imagination. 'The Quality of Wellbeing Scale' is a scientific study that measures the level of wellbeing in your life. In this study, Meniere's is comparable to very ill adults with a life threatening illness such as Cancer or Aids. This was established when Meniere's sufferers were not even having acute episodes! When having acute attacks, the Quality of Wellbeing for Meniere's sufferers is closer to a non-institutionalized Alzheimer's patient, an Aids victim, or a Cancer patient... six days before death. The research quantifies that Meniere's sufferers lose 43.9% from the optimum wellbeing position of normal people. They say Meniere's sufferers are the most severely impaired non-hospitalized patients studied so far. This score reflects major impairment in mobility, physical activity, social activity and clear thinking patterns.

I have to mention these very unpleasant factors, because living in a knowledge vacuum about Meniere's does create confusion and a loss of perspective. This information puts experiences of depression, mobility, social difficulties and clear thinking into perspective. Most Meniere's patients are in the significantly depressed category. So if you think you are having difficulty with Meniere's it's not surprising. If you recognize any symptoms of stress and depression, on the next few pages, help yourself to some further reading.

MAKE GOOD HEALTH COME TRUE

Back to the famous Frenchman Coué. He recommended to patients that they repeat to themselves, when they wake in the morning, twenty times, the now famous phrase, 'Every day in every way I am getting better and better.' Taking a leaf out of his book I did the same every morning.

Coué also encouraged his patients to get into a comfortable, relaxed position before sleep. First to close their eyes and relax all the muscles in the body. As soon as they started to doze off into the semiconscious stage he suggested they introduce into their minds any de-

sired idea..for example 'I am going to be relaxed tomorrow.' This is a way of bridging your
conscious and unconscious minds and allowing
your unconscious to make a positive healing
thought come true.

VISUALIZE THIS HEALING MEDITATION

'Imagine a white healing light shining down on the top of your head. See the light and feel it surrounding your head. Then see the white light fill the inside of your head; cleansing, healing and repairing. Now the light spreads through your entire body. Healing and repairing. Imagine yourself healthy, strong, revitalized and now with renewed energy. Feel a balanced come back into life life. Now you can do what you want to do. Feel renewed.'

This is one example of visual healing. You can use this as a model or create your own healing imagery. Practise at least one healing visualization everyday.

BOOKS TO READ FOR ANXIETY.

Books:

Wherever You Go, There You Are: Mindfulness Meditation In Everyday Life.

- Jon Kabat-Zinn

Full Catastrophe Living (Revised Edition): Using the Wisdom of Your Body and Mind to Face Stress, Pain, and Illness

- Hanh, Thich Nhat and Kabat-Zinn,

Healing Visualizations: Creating Health Through Imagery

- Gerald Epstein

Anxiety, Phobias, and Panic

- Reneau Z. Peurifoy

BOOKS TO READ FOR DEPRESSION, POWERLESSNESS, HOPELESSNESS, POOR SELF-ESTEEM.

Books:

The Depression Cure: The 6-Step Program to Beat Depression without Drugs

- Dr Steve Ilardi

Self-Esteem: A Proven Program of Cognitive Techniques for Assessing, Improving, and Maintaining Your Self-Esteem...

- Fanning, Patrick and McKay, Matthew

The Mindful Way Through Depression: Freeing Yourself from Chronic Unhappiness (Book & CD)

- Williams, Mark

BOOKS TO READ FOR ANGER, RESENTMENT, IRRITABILITY, OBSESSION AND FEAR.

Books:

Calming Your Anxious Mind: How Mindfulness and Compassion Can Free You from Anxiety, Fear, and Panic

- Brantley, Jeffrey and Kabat-Zinn, Jon

Time Management and Goal Setting: The Relaxation and Stress Reduction Workbook Chapter Singles (The New Harbinger Self-Help Essentials)

- Martha Davis, Elizabeth Robbins Eshelman, Matthew McKay

Mindfulness for Beginners: Reclaiming the Present Moment--and Your Life

- Kabat-Zinn, Jon

BOOKS TO READ FOR FATIGUE, BEING TIRED ALL THE TIME, MUSCLE TENSION.

Books:

The Healing Power of the Breath: Simple Techniques to Reduce Stress and Anxiety, Enhance Concentration, and Balance

- Brown MD, Richard and Patricia, MD Gerbarg

Breathing: The Master Key to Self Healing (The Self Healing Series)

- Andrew Weil

Meditation for Optimum Health: How to Use Mindfulness and Breathing to Heal

- Andrew Weil and Jon Kabat-Zinn

AUTHOR PROLOGUE

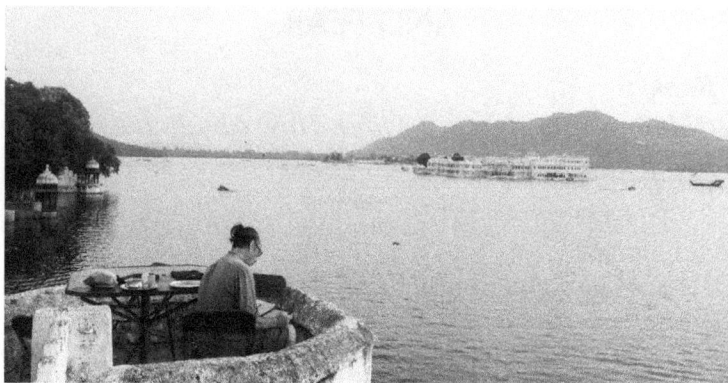

As I have written in my other books, the impact Meniere's has on your life will not always be understood by non-sufferers. I once read that a High Court Judge, a man of the highest social order, publicly stated on record that "Meniere's disease is a mere minor inconvenience." Now, don't you wish that was true! Be aware that the opposite of empathy can be true. Some people have such a lack of understanding towards Meniere's sufferers.

Until non-sufferers understand the impact of Meniere's disease, then sufferers are vulnerable on a physical, mental, emotional and financial level because they may not receive the support necessary to cope. Worse, Meniere's sufferers can run the risk of being financially disadvantaged or even financially ruined by social systems and corporate institutions that should be supportive.

People who suffer from the long term chronic condition of Meniere's lose touch with the possibilities of their potential. We often restrict activities because we feel so bad. We won't extend ourselves and try new things. We find it difficult and become fearful of extending our limits. Fear makes cowards of us all. And we cease to discover what we may be capable of doing.

Health is the most important factor in your life. Health is the real wealth. Money comes and goes, but good health matters more than the size of your wallet. Aim for a simple, uncomplicated life. Don't forget to give yourself personal time and personal space. Make time each day just for you.

Life is on your side.
Go out and live it.

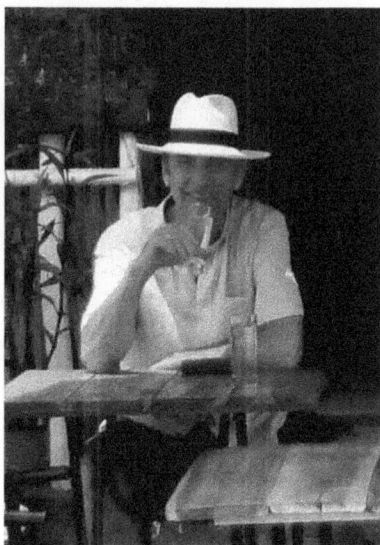

ABOUT THE AUTHOR

At the height of his business career and aged just forty-six, he suddenly became acutely ill. He was diagnosed with Meniere's disease, but the full impact of having Meniere's disease was to come later. He was to lose not only his health, but his career and financial status as he knew it. He began to lose all hope that he would fully recover a sense of well-being. But it was his personal spirit and desire to get back to normal that made him not give up to a life of Meniere's symptoms of severe vertigo, dizziness and nausea.

He decided that you can't put a limit on anything in life. Rather than letting Meniere's disease get in the way of recovery, he started to focus on what to do about overcoming Meniere's disease.

These days life is different for the Author. He is a fit active man who has no symptoms of Meniere's disease except for hearing loss and tinnitus in one ear. He does not take any medication. All the physical activities he enjoys these days require a high degree of balance and equilibrium: snowboarding, surfing, hiking, windsurfing and weightlifting. Things he started to do while suffering with Meniere's disease to help his balance.

'If you want to experience a marked improvement in health you can't wait until you feel well to start. You must begin to improve your health now, even though you don't feel like it.'

With a smile and a sense of humor, the Author pens himself as Meniere Man, because, as he says, Meniere's disease is the one thing that changed his life dramatically. The Author is now a best selling author, designer and artist. He is married to a Poet and Essayist. They have two adult children. He enjoys the sea, cooking, travel, photography, nature and the great company of family, friends and his beloved rescue dog Bella.

BELLA

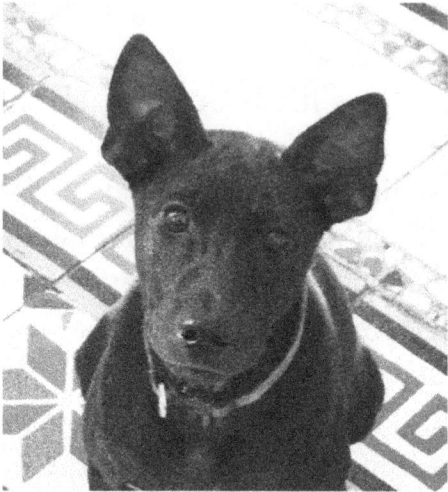

ADDITIONAL INFORMATION

This book and other Meniere Man books are available worldwide from international booksellers and local bookstores.

MENIERE SUPPORT NETWORKS

Meniere's Society (UNITED KINGDOM)
www.menieres.org.uk
Meniere's Society Australia (AUSTRALIA)
info@menieres.org.au
The Meniere's Resource & Information Centre (AUSTRALIA)
www.menieres.org.au
Healthy Hearing & Balance Care (AUSTRALIA)
www.healthyhearing.com.au
Vestibular Disorders association (AUSTRALIA
)www.vestibular .org
The Dizziness and Balance Disorders Centre (AUSTRALIA)
www.dizzinessbalancedisorders.com
Meniere's Research Fund Inc   (AUSTRALIA)
www.menieresresearch.org.au
Australian Psychological Society APS (AUSTRALIA)
www.psychology.org.au
Meniere's Disease Information Center (USA)
www.menieresinfo.com
Vestibular Disorders Association (USA)
www.vestibular.org
BC Balance and Dizziness Disorders Society (CANADA)
www.balanceand dizziness.org
Hearwell (NEW ZEALAND)
www.hearwell.co.nz
WebMD.
www.webmd.com
National Institute for Health
www.medlineplus.gov
Mindful Living Program
www.mindfullivingprograms.com
Center for Mindfulness
www. umassmed.edu.com

MENIERE MAN BOOKS

MENIERE MAN
AND THE ASTRONAUT

THE
SELF HELP
BOOK FOR
MENIERE'S
DISEASE

**It's the only positive, yet real account
I've read, of what it's really like.**

- L. Forrester.(UK)

PAGE ADDIE PRESS. UNITED KINGDOM. AUSTRALIA

MENIERE MAN

LIVING THE SYMPTOM FREE LIFE - WELL OVER FIFTEEN YEARS

Let's
Get Better

**HOW TO GET OVER MENIERE'S
WITH MY MENIERE SURVIVOR'S GUIDE**

PAGE ADDIE PRESS

MENIERE MAN
AND THE FILM DIRECTOR

THE
SELF HELP
BOOK FOR
MENIERE'S
VERTIGO

*This book really helped me get up
and get moving. It helped give me the
desire to get on with life.*

- CDW

PAGE ADDIE PRESS
UNITED KINGDOM. AUSTRALIA

MENIERE MAN
IN THE KITCHEN

RECIPES THAT HELPED ME GET OVER MENIERE'S DISEASE

Delicious nutritious low salt recipes from our family kitchen

PAGE ADDIE PRESS. UNITED KINGDOM AUSTRALIA

MENIERE MAN
IN THE KITCHEN

BOOK 2
RECIPES THAT HELPED ME GET OVER MENIERE'S

DELICIOUS LOW SALT RECIPES
FROM OUR FAMILY KITCHEN

PAGE ADDIE PRESS. UNITED KINGDOM. AUSTRALIA

MENIERE MAN
IN THE HIMALAYAS

COOKING LOW SALT CURRIES IN THE KITCHENS OF INDIA

LOW SALT CURRIES

PAGE ADDIE PRESS. UNITED KINGDOM. AUSTRALIA

MENIERE MAN
IN THE KITCHEN

COOKING
FOR
MENIERE'S
THE
LOW SALT
WAY

ITALIAN

OUR MUCH LOVED ITALIAN
LOW SALT FAMILY RECIPES

PAGE ADDIE PRESS. UNITED KINGDOM. AUSTRALIA

MENIERE MAN

AND THE BUTTERFLY

The
Meniere
Effect

HOW TO MANAGE
THE LIFE CHANGING
EFFECTS OF
MENIERE'S

**KEEPING LIFE POSITIVE THROUGH
THE DIFFICULT TIMES OF MENIERE'S**

PAGE ADDIE PRESS. UNITED KINGDOM. AUSTRALIA

MENIERE MAN

VERTIGO
VERTIGO

ABOUT VERTIGO
ABOUT DIZZINESS
AND WHAT YOU CAN DO
ABOUT IT

MENIERE MAN
GUIDED MEDITATION. VOICED BY MENIERE MAN

Let's
Get Better
Relaxing Healing
Meditation